Autoimmune Disease Diet:

Natural Way to Cure Autoimmune Disorder, Recovery of Immune System and Chronic Pain Relief

By

Valerie Alston

Table of Contents

Introduction 5
Chapter 1. Diagnosis and Manifestations 7
Chapter 2. Treatments for Autoimmune Disease 10
Chapter 3. Nutrition 15
    What to avoid 15
    What to eat 16
Chapter 4. Rest, Exercises and Stress 24
Final Words 31
Thank You Page 32

Autoimmune Disease Diet: Natural Way to Cure Autoimmune Disorder, Recovery of Immune System and Chronic Pain Relief

By Valerie Alston

© Copyright 2014 Valerie Alston

Reproduction or translation of any part of this work beyond that permitted by section 107 or 108 of the 1976 United States Copyright Act without permission of the copyright owner is unlawful. Requests for permission or further information should be addressed to the author.

This publication is designed to provide accurate and authoritative information in regard to the subject matter covered. This work is sold with the understanding that the publisher is not engaged in rendering legal, accounting, or other professional services. If legal advice or other expert assistance is required, the services of a competent professional person should be sought.

First Published, 2014

Printed in the United States of America

Introduction

Full of wonder is one description that fits the nature of the human body. How a newborn, who had never been hungry, instinctively knows that feeding from his or her mother's breasts will satisfy his or her need, is one proof of the amazing design of the human body. Among other astounding pieces of evidence of such beauty is how the body is programmed to defend itself from danger internally, without you having to know it.

Immunity is the condition in which there are adequate biological 'soldiers' in your body, in both in quality and in quantity. These defenses function to fight infection, illness, or other uninvited biological attack. It is also defined as the body's competence to protect itself from harmful microorganisms from getting into it. How the body has its own solutions to such dangers, without you even commanding it to. But, is it not too good to be true? Could there not be a glitch somewhere?

The system of immune responses of an organism against its own (auto) cells and tissues is known as autoimmunity. The immune system's losing of the capacity to distinguish the body's own proteins from those of foreign matter, leads to a condition called an autoimmune disease. Signs and symptoms of this condition are caused by the immune system attacking its own body's cells. Yes, your immune system allows itself to attack some of your cells as well. Although more popularly viewed as anomalous, such response is also seen as an integral part of your immune system. However, diseases labeled as autoimmune may result from such phenomenon, including diabetes mellitus (type I), rheumatic heart disease, multiple sclerosis, systemic lupus erythematosus, hyperthyroidism (Grave's disease), hypothyroidism and Celiac disease, among many others. Such diseases are associated with risk factors such as sex, environment and genetics.

Chapter 1. Diagnosis and Manifestations

Diagnosing an autoimmune disease involves both looking into the signs and symptoms one is manifesting, and identifying the antibodies the body is producing. There are several tests taken from patients who are suspected of having such problem, some of which are autoantibody tests, c-reactive protein, antinuclear antibody test, erythrocyte sedimentation rate, and complete blood count.

Autoantibody tests, any of the handful of tests that look for rather specific antibodies to the body's own tissues are one of the diagnostic measures for autoimmune diseases. Further, another test used is called the antinuclear antibody test, a type of autoantibody examination that searches for the antibodies that attack the nuclei of the cells in the body. Since inflammation is a major concern in autoimmune problems, C-reactive protein (CRP) and erythrocyte sedimentation rate (ESR) are two other tests used to help diagnose severity of one's condition. The former's results, when elevated, indicates inflammation throughout the body, while the latter indirectly measures how much inflammation there is the body. Also, a complete blood count (CBC), which measures the number of red and white blood cells in the blood is also facilitated, since varying values are expected when the immune system is hyped.

While cues from diagnostic examinations are used to come up with a proper diagnosis, so are data coming from the results of a physical examination done to a patient. Doctors are looking for the common signs and symptoms of autoimmune diseases. These include joint or muscle pain, weakness or tremor; insomnia, weight loss, rapid heartbeat or heat tolerance; sun-sensitivity, recurrent rashes or hives, a butterfly-shaped rash across your nose and cheeks; difficulty focusing, feeling tired or fatigues, weight gain or cold tolerance; Hair loss or white patches on your skin or inside your mouth; abdominal pain, mucus or blood in you stool, or mouth ulcers; numbness and tingling sensation in limbs; dry eyes, mouth or skin; and multiple miscarriages or blood clots.

Once the diagnostic test results and physical manifestations are sorted and analyzed, a clearer diagnostic may be made, leading to a decision on which specific treatments are suitable for the patient.

Chapter 2. Treatments for Autoimmune Disease

The autoimmune condition arises through abnormal reactions of the immune system. Here, the patient's immune system is activated against its own body's own proteins, as it fails to recognize such as its own. As such, the most critical goal of managing autoimmune diseases is controlling inflammation, by activation of anti-inflammatory genes and the suppression of inflammatory genes. Generally, the traditional medical management for autoimmune diseases includes anti-inflammatory, immunosuppressive, and palliative treatments.

Anti-inflammatory treatment. The goal of anti-inflammatory approach is to counter the inflammatory response of the body, which also leads to manifestations of the particular autoimmune diseases. Two common classifications of drugs that are ordered to decrease discomfort brought about by the stimulation of the inflammatory process, are non-steroidal anti-inflammatory medications (NSAIDS), and Corticosteroid anti-inflammatory medications.

However, medications are not only the means by which inflammation is controlled in autoimmune disease.

Finding what causes inflammation is considered by some doctors as ultimate way to control inflammation, as treating the root cause and stopping it from prevailing stops the need for such body response, and in turn, their resulting manifestations. Taking down the stimulus for inflammation is more important than addressing the signs and symptoms (and then what?). It is like addressing the fire, not the smoke. This being said, the anti-inflammatory approach in treating autoimmune diseases is not entirely drug-related.

Immunosuppresion. On the other hand, the concept of immunosuppression is quite self-explanatory. Since the immune system becomes active during an autoimmune response, which damages certain tissues in the human body, an approach to calm the system is ideally sought to lessen such damage, hence reducing the consequent signs and symptoms. Some of the immunosuppressive treatment for autoimmune disease range from the use of immunosuppressive drug therapy, to recent research on autologous hematopoietic stem cell transformation. Both and all other strategies to manage autoimmune diseases through immunosuppression involve an act that reduces the activation or efficacy of the immune system. Treatments as such cannot be taken for long periods of time, as doing so increases the risk for severe infections and cancer.

The palliative approach. Further, using a palliative approach aims to reduce the effects or symptoms of the disease, without really curing it. Autoimmune diseases are incurable, but can be controlled, and so managing the presenting signs and symptoms towards more comfortable living is sought. Palliative care is actually a multidisciplinary approach, which focuses on providing patients with relief from the symptoms, pain, physical stress, and mental stress of an illness, regardless of diagnosis. The goal of such is to improve quality of life, considering the incurable nature of the disease, as well as the achievability of controlling its effects. Palliative therapies are given without curative intent, when no cure can be expected, although is also used along with curative or aggressive therapies in some other cases.

Palliative care in autoimmune diseases, as in other cases, is provided by a team of doctors, nurses, and other health care professionals who work together to provide further support.

Lifestyle modification

Considering that the goal of treatment for patients with an autoimmune disease is managing inflammation, it is worth remembering that anything that causes, triggers or worsens inflammation is to be avoided, if not stopped – from physical activities, sleeping hours and lifestyle, to medications and diet. Given that autoimmune diseases have no cure, it is essential to prevent it from worsening. What can be avoided must be avoided now.

While nutrient deficiency has been identified as one of the most significant aggravating factors in autoimmune problems, balancing rest and activity and managing stress, are also essential in reducing the risks for their symptoms' worsening. Basically, it refers to lifestyle.

The good thing about managing autoimmune problems is that although there currently is no known cure for it, aside from that options for medical approaches are available, the person himself of herself may be in control of his or her body, through lifestyle modification. Basically, doing so has something to do with relaxing the self, avoiding negativity; it is basically loving, and being responsible for oneself – something that should come out rather naturally – and that is what makes it even better. You get to go back to the basic, and become less unhealthy. Further, you get to empower yourself to become more consciously in control of your own body – what a way to enhance intrapersonal relations.

Chapter 3. Nutrition

To reiterate, nutrient deficiency is a significant contributing factor in what autoimmune diseases do to the body. To address this, it is obvious that something is to be done with what is lacking in one's diet. But first, what is needed must first be understood.

Research has found a clear connection between certain Neolithic foods – grains, breads, potatoes, beans and dairy, among others – and some autoimmune diseases. By omitting this kind of foods, many people with autoimmune disease have experienced relief from most of the symptoms of such kind of problem.

On the other hand, availability of foods that strengthen the immune system should be taken advantage of, while avoiding what further harms the body.

What to avoid

Generally, any food that may cause irritation or any degree of allergic reaction, causing inflammation, should not be consumed by a person with autoimmune problems.

As for what is to be avoided completely, the following must be written down and placed on the fridge.

Eggs, nuts and seeds, including cocoa, coffee and seed-based spices, have no room in the kitchen.

Potatoes, tomatoes, eggplants, peppers, and other nightshades, are neither welcome in the alimentary tract.

Grains and legumes not be attempted to be taken in.

Dairy products of any kind, should not be consumed.

Aspirin, ibuprofen, and other non-steroidal anti-inflammatory drugs or NSAIDs cannot be administered to the same.

Refined sugars, excessive fructose, non-nutritive sweeteners, emulsifiers, thickeners, and other food additives should be scrapped of the grocery list.

Alcohol, although some may contain probiotics is never healthy for persons with autoimmune diseases.

What to eat

While there is a longer list of foods to be avoided, some nutrients are considered helpful for persons with autoimmune problems. These include vitamin D, omega-3 fatty acids, probiotics, and antioxidants. What follow are descriptions for each nutrient, as well as its sources.

Vitamin D

What it is: Vitamin D belongs to a group of vitamins that are fat-soluble. Sufficient levels of vitamin D aide in the regulation of the immune system, as they are chemically related to steroids, with T and B cells having receptors for it.

What to get it from: Sunlight exposure allows you to absorb vitamin D. If you do not spend enough time in the sun – at least 20 to 25 minutes, you may not get enough. Common vitamin D-rich foods include fatty fish, liver, and fortified orange juice. However, although one of the most convenient was to get vitamin D is egg yolk, as well as fortified milk, since its presence can be found in so many recipes, these are not recommended food for persons with autoimmune disease.

Fatty fish coming from salmon, trout, mackerel, tuna and eel, is a good source of vitamin D. Aside from getting vitamin D, you also get to have omega-3 fatty acids.

Omega-3 fatty acids

What it is: Omega-3 is composed of polyunsaturated fatty acids, which, when consumed adequately, may counteract the effects of arachidonic acid, a kind of unsaturated fatty acid contributing to the symptoms of autoimmune diseases. It also inhibits the production of cytokines that cause the physiological symptoms of depression, which are also inflammatory and autoimmune in nature. Omega-3-rich foods are best eaten raw, as the nutrient is easily damaged by oxygen, light and heat.

What to get it from: Foods rich in this nutrient that may be consumed by persons with autoimmune diseases include beef, wild rice, canola oil, fish, fish oils, green leafy vegetables. Although flax seed and flax seed oil, beans, dairy of pasture-raised animals, enriched eggs, and walnuts and walnut oil are excellent sources of omega-3, they are to be avoided because seed is not good for a person with autoimmune disease.

Wild rice, that which is grown in farms, being grass more than rice, is richer in omega-3, and is healthier for persons with autoimmune problems compared with brown or white rice, which are grains. In frying, consider using canola oil. The fish and fish oils mentioned earlier are also good sources of omega-3.

Probiotics

What it is: Good bacteria are what probiotics are often referred to. Including them in the diet of persons with autoimmune diseases helps strengthen one's immune system, and aides in the absorption of essential vitamins and minerals. Containing live bacteria, this preparation is a dietary supplement that is taken orally to restore beneficial bacteria to the body.

What to get it from: Foods rich in probiotics include most that is fermented food and beverage. Among such are kimchi, a spicy vegetable side dish, which is usually served in every meal in Korea, Kombucha, a refreshing beverage made out of sweetened black tea. Some yogurt products, fermented, also contain live and active cultures, but just like fermented beer, are not good for persons with autoimmune disease because it is a milk product.

Antioxidants

What it is: Linked with beta-carotene or vitamin C, antioxidants inhibit oxidation or reaction promoted by oxygen, peroxides or 'free radicals', damaged cells that can be problematic. The danger with free radicals is that when they are on attack, they injure cells in their DNA, creating the seed for disease. The role of antioxidants in protecting your body is to keep the free radicals under control, or to stop the damaging, disease-causing chain reaction that they trigger.

What to get it from: Although contained in almost any food supplement being marketed in the present, antioxidants are still good taken from natural sources. Again, nuts and berries are great sources of antioxidants, but they belong to the list of foods that are to be generally avoided in autoimmune diseases.

Dark-colored grapes contain phytochemicals, which can boost the immune system. They also contain vitamin C and selenium. Dark green vegetables are also excellent sources of antioxidants. Not only do they have a high content of calcium, magnesium, potassium, and vitamins A, E, and C, they are also loaded with antioxidant phytochemicals to help regulate the immune system.

All in all, the following food should be eaten more:
Organ meat and offal, around five times a week
Fish and shellfish, around three times a week, except if hypersensitive to such
Vegetable of all kinds – green, colourful, cruciferous and sea, except for algae (immune stimulators), around eight to 14 cups a day
Grass-fed, pasture raised quality meats (and fat)
Fruit, maximum of 20g daily
Fermented vegetables or fruit
Glycine-rich foods

How the meal plan should look like

Any food plan employing a balance in any of the aforementioned foods is good to fight the effects of autoimmune disease. Again, you may not be able to cure it, but you have the power to manage it – not only through medical treatments, but more importantly, in an aspect you are more hands on – your diet. Maintaining three to four meals that look like the following meal plan prototype will be a good balance. This may appear or even actually be difficult to adjust to for many, but it may help to remember what symptoms and complications are being prevented from worsening. It is also of greatest significance to be faithful with the therapeutic diet recommended.

Lean protein: chicken, beef, fish, or offal, around 4 to 8 ounces

Steamed, half-cooked, or raw leaves: dark or colourful

Probiotic food: kimchi, kombucha or supplements

Bone broth, one cup

Fruit, maximum of 20g per day (fractions thereof in to be included in different meals)

Overview to simple recipes

For simple cooking, you may want to consider stir-frying vegetables with some organ meat to supply you with protein, keeping in mind only the allowed spices. It is best preferred half-cooked. If you prefer raw veggies, then you may want to prepare a recipe of vegetable and fruit salad in considerably large servings, carefully choosing your rainbow leaves, with fresh fruit such as grapes or apples – depending on which suits your taste best. You may include in your salad some leftover meat, offal or fish to add on some protein. In case you are up for more protein in one of your meals, make sure to partner it with some kimchi to make your dining experience more exciting.

Chapter 4. Rest, Exercises and Stress

While it has been repeatedly emphasized that diet is highly influential in controlling the symptoms of autoimmune diseases, the fact that there are also other factors which you can manage, as much as you are in control of what you eat, cannot be isolated. You can command your body and implement the same commands on dealing with rest, exercise and stress.

Ensuring an Adequate Rest

For people belonging to a certain age bracket, sleep is far from being their best friend. It has never seemed to be on their side, and so they would rather be 'productive', and do some more – worse, with a cup of coffee at hand. Irrespective of age, sex, condition, lifestyle or anything, sleep is supposed to be always healthy at an average of eight hours in every 24 hours of your life. Your body, even at normal circumstances, needs to pause and recharge, in order to maintain a functional state. This is how you take good care of your body.

Aside from boosting your immune system, sleep in acceptable amount, also speeds up your metabolism, gives you a longer attention span, puts you in a better disposition, allows you to look more attractive, gives you better memory, and lengthens your lifespan. But what if normal sleep is really not attainable for you?

Sleep is supposed to be normal. A human body is entitled to rest. In fact, it is supposed to rest. However, due to certain direct and indirect interruptions with the circadian rhythm, or your body clock, sleep sometimes becomes difficult to achieve. How to address this is of course, trying to determine what keep you awake. If it's the environment, there must be a need to rearrange the room, or get a better lamp, or just turn off the lights. If it's a thought that keeps running in your mind, you might need to settle it during the day, before you hit the sack. If it just works better for you to take naps during the day, you probably need to work on rest schedules so you can have enough.

There is a growing list of hacks on how to get yourself to sleep. Pick out the ones that work for you, so you can get that eight-hour rest, strengthen your immunity, and be more healthy.

Exercising regularly

Studies say that at least 30 minutes of physical activity everyday can help control weight, combat diseases, improve your mood, boost your energy, promote better sleep, and provide recreation, among others.

A balance between rest and activity is always crucial in trying to achieve, if not maintain homeostasis in the body. Homeostasis refers to a state balance and harmony among the different organs and systems comprising an organism – in your case, a human body. A life full of sleep, naps, rest and lying around is a lazy person's life – not at all healthy. While a good amount of sleep is recommended to people with autoimmune problems, adequate exercise spurs it up to productivity.

Reducing stress

Stress is a situation wherein you experience mental anxiety or discomfort, usually because of certain stimuli, called stressors which are usually 'bad'. Stress in medical perspective, however, is not always bad, per se, as stimuli that cause a person to get excited are considered as stressors just the same. How could winning the lottery be something you would like to 'reduce' (as per 'stress reduction')? How could seeing your loved one be something you would want to get over with? Considering both perspectives though, it can be understood that stress indeed causes anxiety. It in fact, causes tension, only, stressors should not be limited to just 'problems'.

Bad or good even, any amount of stress significantly affects your health, whether or not you are eating the right food, you have adequate amount of sleep, or you are exercising enough. As some would say, stress, not the cancer, would kill a person suffering from the manifestations of a terminal disease. In dealing with stress, whether a stressor makes us worried or thrilled, it would be helpful for your health if you learn how to manage it properly and effectively. The list of ways to manage stress should encompass how to live a healthy and happy life. It covers many aspects from the diet, exercise and sleep, to decision making and spirituality. It is too great to reduce its discussion to mere overview, but the following practical tips should help you.

The steps

First, you need to be aware of where the anxiety comes from. What stresses you out? What is the root cause of what makes you worry? Did you panic because your boss is calling you on the phone? Is it because of the mere sight of his name on your mobile's screen, or is it because of fear you might have done something again? Now where is this fear coming from? Have you done something in the past that you haven't gotten over with? Try to dig in the deepest possible for you to be able to understand the innermost root cause of this seemingly superficial stressor.

Second, realize and analyze what you are and are not capable of. Once you have identified you most basic stressor, what can you do to address it? Which among your strengths can you utilize in order to eradicate this issue? Since you have touched on your strengths, what about your weaknesses? What are the areas you need to work on?

Third, avoid what stresses you out. It always takes self-awareness to be able to work on a solution to anything. Now that you have laid down your cards to yourself, what strategies can you employ to get rid of the things that trigger you to be unnecessarily concerned? Can you prevent yourself from having to face another stressor that you have not learned to deal with yet? How do you differentiate being concerned from getting worried? How do you intend to choose your battles?

Fourth, do what makes you happy. While avoiding what pins you down, it's time to arm yourself with positivity. What makes you happy? What keeps you peaceful? What calms you down? Be it outdoor activities, reading a book, doing a movie marathon, writing a dissertation, playing with the dog, singing songs or meditating, go ahead and get those endorphins going. With this, stay healthy. Eat well. Be faithful with your diet. Exercise regularly. Have enough sleep. Maintain good dealings with friends. Stay away from illness. Be healthy holistically. And be happy doing it.

Final Words

Complicated as it is, the human body is indeed full of wonder. It sometimes requires you to aide it to function at its fullest, but has its way of amazing you. Although autoimmune diseases truly put one in a rather difficult state, what you should focus on is that the beauty of the make-up of the human body includes the truth that although part of it seems to be on an autopilot mode, you own it, and can take control.

Again, there is no known cure for problems caused by autoimmunity. But this does not mean there is nothing you can do. You can not only manage the symptoms of autoimmune diseases, you can also reduce the risks of its complications. Some adjustment in lifestyle and diet may be difficult, but will do the trick. After all, it is your body.

Thank You Page

I want to personally thank you for reading my book. I hope you found information in this book useful and I would be very grateful if you could leave your honest review about this book. I certainly want to thank you in advance for doing this.